A GUIDE TO DECEPTION: THE INSANITY TO HUMAN SANITY

(PROLOGUE)

A woman working at a Jewelry store disheartoningly informs her manager that she has cancer, and needs more vacation time for her upcoming surgeries. Her manager allows her as much vacation time as she needs. Suddenly, diamond rings go missing. The manager cannot figure out who is stealing the diamond rings, and costing his company thousands of dollars in loss. So, he hires a detective. The detective informs the manager that all evidence is pointing towards the woman with cancer as the culprit.

With a heavy heart, the manager asks the woman if she is taking jewelry from the inventory. The woman cries tears of shock in front of him. She tells him she has cancer, she is dying, and she simply wants to spend her last few months at the job she loves and with her daughter. With a heavy and very guilty heart, the manager apologizes for asking and tells the detective to dig deeper.

"It can't be her," said the manager.

The detective searches more extensively than before, and comes across a video that shows the woman with cancer slipping a diamond ring into her back pocket.

The next time the woman comes into work, the manager brings her into his office. Since she is sick, he takes pity on her. He lets her know that he is aware that she is the thief, that he is hurt that she lied to him, but allows her the option of returning all the stolen jewelry. If she does this, he says, all will be forgiven. She returns only one diamond ring and claims that she did not steal the rest. She cries, she says that she has cancer and she is dying and she just wanted to leave some money so *her daughter could go to college. The manager feels sorry for her again, fires her, (without reporting her to the police) and lets her go home.*

Three years later, he runs into the woman at a very high-end restaurant having dinner with an attractive man. Surprised, he steps forward and looks at her glittering heels, her designer handbag, her bright blonde hair and her delicate makeup. He approaches her, and she immediately recognizes him.

"You look very healthy. I am very glad you seem to be feeling better," says her former manager

The woman smiles back at him. He immediately recognizes the diamond necklace she has placed around her neck.

"I never was sick, sir. It was too easy."

This text emphasizes the nature of humans and discusses the variations of innate impulses; it further discusses the morality associated with human nature along with human beliefs and cognition. I will not only accentuate the underlying's of deceptive behavior but I will more importantly silver the linings of so-called "normal" behavior by delving into the consciousness of an individual. In simpler terms, I will prove to you that just as the woman relied on the manager's emotions in order to manipulate him, the human brain relies on your own emotions in order to manipulate you. Surely the darkest of devious skills delves from the purest of human souls.

DEDICATED TO

SAMRANA HUSAIN AND ANWAR HUSAIN

(MAMA AND PAPA)

MY SUCCESS IS BY MY PARENTS

CONTENTS:

i. THE BRAIN, OR THE MIND? DOES FAITH CONSTITUTE KNOWLEDGE?

ii. PSYCHOLOGICAL MYTHS

iii. ILLOGICAL LOGIC

iv. WHY DO GOOD PEOPLE, DO BAD THINGS?

v. GOOD OR BAD?

vi. BIAS

vii. EVIL (JEALOUSY, GOSSIP, AND LYING)

viii. DETECTING A LIAR

ix. DETECTING A PSYCHOPATH

x. DETECTING A THIEF

xi. THE ILLUSION OF BEAUTY

xii. THE ILLUSION OF LOVE

xiii. HOW TO MAKE PEOPLE LIKE YOU

THE BRAIN, OR THE MIND? DOES FAITH CONSTITUTE KNOWLEDGE?

Let me provide you with three facts that are simply irrefutable: the human brain controls our nervous system, it keeps us working (walking, talking, thinking, breathing), and it is so complex it consists of over one *billion* neurons. Now let me provide you with a rather popular opinion: the functioning brain is not identical to the mind. This particular belief is known as dualism. The reasoning behind this concept is solely based on mystery; since the mind cannot be explained without going hand in hand with the brain, dualists instead assume that the mind is created by material that we cannot see (immaterial), such as a persons' soul, or spirit. This soul can live on without the brain, which justifies the dualist belief of the afterlife. The view of

dualism holds that we, as humans, do have a spirit and body and that they are two separate components of us. Contrarily, those that believe the opposite are referred to as materialists. Materialism is a view that says humans are made up solely of material and have no non material part like a soul or spirit. This view holds the stance that the physical aspects of human bodies is highly complex and advanced on its' own. In simpler terms, materialism relies solely on facts that can be proven, rather than trusting the unknown. Dualism is rather unsuitable; since it leans towards religious beliefs and cannot be proved to be true, dualists have a rather difficult time understanding the nature of consciousness.

Imagine a Pediatric surgeon treats a child who just moved here from Kenya. This child has odd purple spots on her foot. Thus, her surgeon infers that the purple spots on her foot came from some sort of disease in Kenya. She has no proof, there is no record of any purple spot diseases in Kenya, and so far it has not seemed to have any sort of detrimental effect on the patient. According to Theodore Schick, a philosopher, to have knowledge, then, we must have adequate evidence, and our evidence is adequate when it puts the proposition in question beyond a reasonable doubt. This surgeon does not have adequate evidence, therefore she is not certain about this disease; she can only make a guess- an educated guess, but a guess nonetheless. Guesses, whether educated or not, are not based on certainty and do not constitute knowledge.

Nevertheless, what actually constitutes knowledge? Dualists may argue that we are not truly certain of almost anything, so certainty cannot constitute knowledge. This argument is defensible. We are not certain of many things. For example, how do I know for sure that I am wearing black sweatpants right now? I could be a schizophrenic patient on the floor of a hospital, hallucinating this entire scenario. In the objective reality that we live in, dualists are safe when assuming that there are few things we are absolutely certain of knowing. However, this basis of uncertainty is not enough to justify the belief of dualism. If certainty does not constitute knowledge, a claim must require enough viable reasons or evidences to prove it beyond a shadow of a doubt. Although doubt is certainly possible, there will come a point by which doubt is no longer *reasonable*. Therefore, evidence constitutes knowledge. To have knowledge, we have to be able to actually establish its' truth beyond a reasonable doubt.

Dualism is the concept that our mind is more than just our brain. This spiritual dimension can only be reinforced by lucidity provided by spiritual holy books, such as the Quran, Bible, or the Torah. So, instead of appealing to logic, dualism appeals to faith, and this is where we must be careful. When speaking about the brain, we must speak in terms of scientific fact. Things become messy when we attempt to pick through the grey areas of life when trying to understanding consciousness. Obviously, it must take evidence to truly prove a claim beyond a shadow of a doubt, which is the opposite of religion. Faith is ordinarily understood as the belief that does not rest on logical proof or material evidence. Let me give you an example. Suppose that I believe it to be true that Mohammad is the messenger of God, and that there is only one God. If you asked me why I trust this to be absolutely accurate, chances are I would tell you that I trust Islam because I feel that it is right in my heart. Chances are, I would advocate the morals set forth in the Quran, and I would talk about how praying gives me a sense of security, so it must be right. There is no hard proof of a single word of this faith, yet hypothetically I am following what the Quran preaches with unwavering doubt. In other words, I believe my religion to be true because I believe in it. In complete honesty, faith trumps all because it is free from doubt. It is, absurdly and entirely, free from doubt, because you cannot doubt an opinion that does not rely on facts. Faith is free from doubt; however, it is inferior to knowledge because it lacks rational justification. Rendered by the RSS, in the case of faith, "the gap between belief and evidence is filled by an act of will- we choose to believe something even though that belief isn't warranted by evidence". So, belief cannot be a source of knowledge. Just because we believe certain things to be true doesn't mean that we are justified in believing it. Faith, in the sense we are considering, is unquestioning, unjustified belief. Unjustified belief cannot constitute knowledge. We can believe that the mind is separate from the body because of a humans' spirit, but that does not make it true. Instead, dualists that use faith to support their argument are only admitting that they do not have any sort of justification. A lack of evidence is no evidence at all.

If I were to give you all the reasons why dualism is inapt and assume that you now realize that materialism must be right because dualism is wrong, I would be contradicting myself. Since adequate evidence constitutes knowledge, let me use reason to prove to you that materialism makes sense beyond a shadow of a doubt. You may remember this news story: a few years ago in Florida, 57-year-old Tammy Sexton was shot in the brain by her husband. She survived, but was reported by her friends to be "not the same Tammy". Obviously, this is because of the bullet that sped through her brain. This bullet altered Sextons' brain to the point where her mind did not function properly anymore. She forgot how to write, read, and eat; she could speak basic words, but her mind had been so badly transformed she barely remembered even her own name. So why did her state of mind alter when her brain was damaged? The answer to this is very simple: *the brain and the mind go hand in hand.* If one is damaged, the other is almost always damaged as well. If the brain was truly a separate component from the mind, and the mind could live on without the brain (such as in the afterlife), then wouldn't Sextons' state of mind be perfectly fine even after being shot in the head?

Materialists argue that by viewing cases of mental disorders it can also be verified that the mind is solely physical matter, and is essentially the same thing as the brain. In 1990, a documentary called *Child of Rage* was made. This particular case was incredibly interesting; *Child of Rage* is about a six-year-old girl named Beth who tries to kill her family and enjoys it. It was stated in this documentary that at two years old, Beth was raped and molested repeatedly by her birth father. According to Beth's therapist, the first three years of a humans' life is when an individual develops feelings of love and trust. Due to her trauma during these ages, Beth never developed this sense of conscious. Her therapy sessions were recorded and played in the documentary, and I can recall one that was rather disturbing. The therapist asked her what she was doing with kitchen knives under her pillow, and Beth tilted her head and smiled. She proceeded to tell him that they were "just in case she wanted to kill someone at night, so that no one could watch her do it in the dark". Mind you, this is a six-year-old child. This little girls' brain did not develop correctly because of her childhood, so her mind did not function with emotions, causing her to lack the ability to feel remorse, much like Ted Bundy or any other famous psychopaths you may have heard of. Once again, the mind worked hand in hand with the brain, rather than separately with the 'soul' or 'spirit' of the girl. If the soul controls the mind which is wholly separate from the brain, why does Beths' mind encourage her to be a stone-cold killer?

A study in 2015 said that approximately 8 out of 10 people in the United States believe that there is an afterlife. Meaning, about 80% of the nation believes that the mind is separate from the brain, and lives on after death. I am not saying this is wrong; I am only pointing out that over half of this country devotionally believes something that cannot be medically, scientifically, or logically proven. It is essentially ridiculous to base a medical standpoint on the human body on something that cannot be medically explained. The afterlife is one of our worlds' greatest mysteries. Religion could very well be a concept made up from some people long ago, who believed that the people in the world need some kind of moral code to follow. Or, it could be very true; things like the Day of Judgment or the afterlife could approach us at any time. We have truly no way of knowing. As humans, not knowing causes us to make assumptions, but we must take the time to accept that there are certain things we cannot make assumptions about. Medicine is science. It is based on hard proof and logic, not ideas and faith. Science is exact.

The purpose of this text is not to prove to you that there is no such thing as ideas such as the afterlife; it is, rather, an attempt at putting in perspective the sheer irrationality to human faith, no matter how true it may feel.

PSYCHOLOGICAL MYTHS:

("COMMON SENSE" BELIEFS THAT ARE NOT TRUE)

1) Catharsis (emotional release, such as venting or punching a punching bag while angry) is a healthy way of relieving anger or sadness. It makes the person feel better, instead of keeping it bottled up.

In 2002, a scholar and Psychologist named Bushman conducted an experiment to test the effectiveness of catharsis. The experimenter made everyone in the experiment angry. Then, the angry people were divided into three groups. One of these groups used a punching bag ten minutes after being made angry. The second group spoke to a counselor and vented about what just happened ten minutes after they were made angry. The third group remained silent, and was not allowed to speak about their anger or express it in any way.

Bushman's results concluded that the people who remained silent about their anger were exponentially better-off than the other two groups after prolonged periods of time. In other words, the people that did not participate in expressing their anger subsided their anger more quickly. I am not discrediting therapy or counseling; there are surely benefits that may come out of speaking about problems. Benefits may include getting advice on a difficult situation, or gaining alternate perspectives other than your own. I am also not saying that it is healthy to bottle every emotion; but, it is surely healthier to train your biases to control your anger over petty scenarios than it is to speak about everything bad that happens to you. In a situation where someone has insulted you or provoked you, you will typically become more and more upset about it the more you talk about it. As long as you are talking about it, you are thinking about it. It is important to remember that if something remains in your mind, **it remains in your heart.** In addition to this, punching a punching bag may be a safer alternative than punching someone in the face, but it may increase your likeliness of resorting to violence or aggression in the case of a future incident. It is an interesting theory to consider- perhaps, that our society could be conditioning us to push a heavier emphasis on our anger than is truly warranted.

2) Human memory is like a recording of what happened.

This is a myth. Our memories are invariably distorted. It is more accurate to say that human memory is like an individually-written movie of what we wanted to happen. Often times, we remember the portions of a scene or day that stood out to us, and this causes us to overlook other details. If you are having a remarkable day- you got the job you wanted and you feel like you are on top of the world. You are likely to remember the way the sunlight was shining while you drove your car or the way your friends laughed at all of your jokes. You may miss out on noticing the one girl out of your group of friends that was upset, or you may miss the portion of time when your friends got tired of hearing you talk about yourself and your job. You were feeling good that day. Memories are more closely related to emotions than they are related to actual incidence.

Here is an example of an incidence where an emotionally-stuffed experience distorts our memory of what happened:

You are walking down the street, and you see a car hit a man. The man falls, and may be dead; and the car moves to the right in what you consider an attempt to drive away. A hit and run. So, you run up to the car, waving your hands, and the driver stops. You call the police. You are an eye-witness to the scene. You literally saw this man trying to drive away with your own eyes, so that is what you confidently tell the police. In reality, the man was not trying to drive away. He was moving towards the right so he could park his car and make sure the guy was alright. However, the shock of the car crash and the adrenaline rushing through your body throughout a high-pressure situation caused you to aggressively and impulsively assume the man was trying to leave, so that is the story your mind sticks with. You are convinced you know what you saw.

In court rooms, we rely on the sighting of eye-witness testimonies, even though we shouldn't. Some may assume that the more confident a witness is of what they saw, the more trustworthy their testimony is. This is not true. It is, in fact, the opposite. On many occasions, the more confident a person is in their sighting of what happened, the more likely they are to ignore details that contradict their belief- details that may add up to the actual truth.

3) People who commit violent crimes are usually mentally ill.

Your common sense tells you that anyone that kills someone, commits mass murder, or participates in a terror attack as a terrorist must be mentally ill. What "normal" person would commit such a crime and not even feel guilty about it, right? **This is false. In a study of crimes committed by people with serious mental disorders, only 7.5% of crimes were directly related to symptoms of a mental disorder.** Notice that when a mentally ill person commits a crime, the media turns somewhat of a blind eye. So, in example, if a schizophrenic patient killed his family, it would be extremely unfortunate, but the media would not emphasize it because the person was mentally ill and this is a socially accepted justification. Also, note that in cases that involve shootings, the popular news channels will often times reflect on the attackers childhood in an attempt to suggest that they are mentally ill. In order to gain a more accurate body of general knowledge, it is time to be more critical of the media. Most shooters, terrorists, and rapists are the seemingly nice, normal people in society with incredibly apt deception skills, which may be the most frightful part of it all.

4) Most domestic violence acts or cases of child abuse are committed by men, not women.

Completely false. In a recent study, it was shown that over 65% of the United States population of adults (18 years and older) believe that most abusers are the men. It is easy to understand why our impulsive minds would lead us to accept this, since men are typically stronger, larger, and more prone to resorting to aggressiveness to solve an issue, whereas women are more prone to participating in relational aggression (ruining one's social standing, gossiping) to let go of anger. The National Intimate Partner and Sexual Violence Survey in the US found that one in four men had experienced physical violence, rape, and/or stalking from a partner (compared to one in three women) and that 83 percent of the violence inflicted on men by partners was done so by women. This is not to diminish the seriousness or scale of the problem of partner abuse by men toward women, but to recognize that there is also a significant, lesser known, issue of women being violent toward men.

5) Smiling makes you happier.

It is commonly understood that if you just smile, you will instantly become a bit happier than you were before. This is not true. One of the most substantial flaws of this myth is it excites the idea that we should be happy all the time, when in reality, it is just not that simple. If merely putting a smile on your face made you a more joyful person, we would have a lot more happiness in this world. However, there one small loophole that may provide this myth with a milligram of truth. If you have a real smile, NOT A FAKE ONE, you are likely to feel better if you were experiencing some identifiable emotions that day (like depression, or anxiety.) So, what I am saying is, it is not smiling that makes people happy, but it is perhaps the small act or happiness that comes along with a real smile that makes a person's mood a little bit more positive.

There are thousands of everyday "common sense" beliefs that are merely inaccurate. I, however, only pointed out five. We believe these myths partly because our mind goes for the easiest option, or the one that makes the most sense. When you are attempting to think about things logically, you may actually be manipulating yourself to believe a story that sounds good or feels right. So, why do we rely on thousands of myths so heavily, without actually looking for the information to constitute knowledge for ourselves?

ILLOGICAL LOGIC

- **VERBAL CLAIMS:**

Word of mouth is dangerous. When an individual makes a statement repeatedly, that does not make it valid in any way. However, hearing a statement made over and over again in confidence may make it *sound* true. For example, consider the recent attacks on the media made by the current President Donald Trump. President Trump has repeated the phrase "fake news" countless times in speeches, interviews, and on social media platforms such as Twitter. Though it may be true that the media is incredibly flawed and/or bias at times, and often edited to make a good story or to gain viewers, that is not the point. Many US citizens have come to discredit media as a whole because of the one phrase that Trump repeats: fake news. Logically, though it usually is biased, news channels are among the most accessible components of free speech that the American people rely on. If Trump said "fake news" once or twice, this comment may be ignored. However, the way he adamantly repeats it in confidence that certain news channels are "fake", he has convinced many American people to disrepute news channels entirely.

- INSTANT GRATIFICATION:

We live in an instant-gratification society. In simper terms, this just means that we live in a society that demands quick and easy results. Whether the issue is burning fat or acing an exam, we want a solution that will fix our problem or put our mind to rest quickly. This is why we are likely to believe a claim if it sounds good. For example, pretend you are frustrated over the acne on your face. After trying multiple skin cleansers and creams, you are not seeing very many results. You see an ad that claims that a new cleanser of their brand gets rid of acne in 24 hours, and you are immediately more inclined to purchase it. You wanted a quick fix, so you believed their claim to be true when in reality, they are probably not telling the truth.

- INFERRING CAUSATION FROM CORRELATION:

One of the most basic lessons taught in every Psychology course is that *correlation does not mean causation.* This common misconstrued tendency to believe that if some variable closely relates to another variable it means that variable must be responsible for the other is simply not grounded evidence. For example, you learn that the number of ice cream sales is positively correlated with the number of people diagnosed with depression. This does not mean that if ice cream sales go up, the number of depressed people also must go up. Depressed people are not responsible for ice cream sales going up, they are only a factor that influences the rise in sales.

WHY DO GOOD PEOPLE, DO BAD THINGS?

Close your eyes and imagine a very functional, 1997 world. You own a small home in Texas. Your neighbors are seemingly good neighbors- whatever "good neighbors" means. They don't make too much noise, they work jobs, have a few kids, plant flowers here and there, and live their own separate lives. One day, their youngest son, Nicholas, goes missing. He was only 8 years old, with beautiful blonde hair and spiking blue eyes. You hear the news and your heart skips a beat, but how do you respond? Because when you lose a family member or something tragic happens, that stays with you forever. Death leaves a forever heartache on a person's soul, so how do you fix that? Bring them a casserole, tell them you'll pray for them, give them a hug? There is nothing you can do but shake your head, and wonder, <u>why do bad things happen to good people?</u>

This question is a common one, and certainly a rather uncanny one, because there is no satisfiable answer to it. You can call it God, or fate, or simply just horrible misfortune for why the nice, quiet neighbors lost their little boy out of nowhere, but there is no real response. Now, formulate every related insoluble question we ask whenever something tragic happens. I made a list of three:

1) Why do bad things happen to good people?
2) Why do good things happen to bad people?
3) Why do bad things happen to bad people?

There is no satisfiable answer to any of these questions. Instead, we can scratch all three of these questions and focus on this one:

Why do we act the way that we do after something important happens to us?

To answer this, we must simply consider our typical ranges of emotions. When something happens, it hurts us because it occurs outside the walls of emotions that we are used to experiencing on a daily basis. The same is true when we are happy because something good happens. We are happy merely because the occurrence took place outside our typical range of emotions. Take lottery winners, for example. "Common sense" might tell you that life is set for the lottery winner- they won what everyone wants.

Here is an example where our "common sense" instinct seems to fail us. A gigantic portion of lottery winners end up with a mental illness (such as depression), ruining relationships built prior to the big win, and more than half of them end up losing their money within the first three years.

Money was never the key to happiness, anyways.

To understand why we act the way that we do, we must first understand why we react the way that we do. I would say that our actions are simply an execution of our reactions. To understand what I mean, take the example of Larry Nassar, the pedophile doctor who abused multiple girls who were gymnasts (2018). The father of two girls who were abused by Nassar stood in the court room to testify against him. As you can imagine, the father's reaction to this man was obviously not a good one. Disgust, anger, rage- all reactions to the inhumane and violating actions preformed on his daughters. The father asked for a moment to speak, and asked the judge if, as part of the man's sentencing, if he would be allowed five minutes alone with Nassar. The judge declined his request, as it does not line up with American ethical or legal policies to basically allow a man to beat someone to death. So, the father pushed past security, and did his best to attack the man that attacked his children. An action that exemplifies his reaction: injustice, sadness, anger. Nonetheless, by attacking someone in a court room he is still breaking the law. I asked you earlier why good people do bad things. Define "bad"- isn't it bad that he broke the law? But, in this situation, was it justified?

GOOD OR BAD?

Moreover, common sense lets you know that there is good or bad, pure evil vs. good, and so on. Obviously, a pedophile is evil, right? In order to comprehensively and accurately evaluate people in a critical way that challenges our walls of general thinking, and in order to understand why people react the way that they do, we must understand the phenomenon of the social constructs of good vs. bad. We all draw an imaginary line in our minds to separate the good from the bad. The father of those two victims in my previous example did it before our eyes. He drew the line- touching his daughters was wrong, it was bad- so this man is a bad man. **Please note, that in this passage I am in no way defending the actions of a pedophile. I am simply probing your mind to consider the wirings of the mind of a criminal man, so we can understand why *he* reacted to the young girls in such an inappropriate and illegal manner, so that we can more accurately come to our conclusions about who to blame.** It was easy to understand the angry reaction of the father of the victims, because in our minds, the father is the good person here. The father has the "right" to be angry. But, in order to challenge ourselves, to extend our knowledge past the general realm of comprehension with as little personal bias as possible, we must do our best to understand the involatile actions of a "bad" person. In other words, the challenge I am presenting you with here is to understand someone who you think is evil. After you delve deeper into your beliefs, instead of easily accepting what comes to mind you may find that sometimes what is truly going on may not line up with the beliefs your mother taught you since you were in kindergarten.

Pedophilia is a disease. That is fact- it is categorized as a mental illness. Pedophilic Disorder is a DSM-5 (Diagnostic and Statistical Manual of Mental Disorders, fifth edition), diagnosis assigned to adults (defined as age 16 and up) who have sexual desire for prepubescent children. Any behavioral expression of Pedophilic Disorder is a criminal offense in the United States, Canada, and Europe, as well as most other places in the world.

So, let's put this in perspective. You have a schizophrenic patient. A girl, named Emily. Emily has lived in a mental hospital since her schizophrenia gave rise when she was 20 years old. If you do not know what schizophrenia is, according to the Diagnostic and Statistical Manual of Mental Disorders, Fifth Edition, (DSM-5), to meet the criteria for diagnosis of schizophrenia, the patient must have experienced at least 2 of the following symptoms: delusions, hallucinations, and/or disorganized speech.

Schizophrenia is common in the psychological world as being the one disease that causes patients to lose touch with their sense of reality. Some of them, the more severe cases, live in a different world: they see things that we do not see, and they hear things that we do not believe are there. Emily hallucinates almost all of the time. She believes that the doctors in the hospital are out to get her. There is someone she calls "jimmy". She yells out Jimmy's name during the day and in her sleep. The doctors have put together that she is afraid of Jimmy. Emily believes that Jimmy is trying to kill her, and on multiple occasions, Emily has screeched at her family and her doctors to exit the room while Jimmy was present for her in her own attempt to save their lives. One day, Emily thinks that Jimmy is whispering to her and telling her to kill her mother. Emily refuses, but Jimmy brings in more killers. The whispers get louder and louder, and they turn into screeches. This is torture. She refuses to leave her room because she does not want to kill her mother. One day, her mother comes into her room. Emily cannot take the devilish screams urging her to murder any longer; she grabs the knife that came with her food that day, and slits her mothers throat. As the whispers die down and Jimmy is no longer present, she shifts into reality and is able to comprehend what she just did. She realizes what she has done, and she feels her heart break and throws up at the sight of her own mother's blood.

"Obviously", murder is wrong. The word "obviously" is contradictory in most cases, because most cases are not so simple or obvious to decipher. Murder might be wrong, but in this case, was it excused? Surely, it is not Emily's fault that she ended up killing somebody. It was the diseases' fault. We know that she would not have done this if it were not for the agonizing torture in her head, because once it went away, she realized what she had done, but it was too late. Court rooms would provide her leeway for being legally psychotic, and would lock her up most likely in a more extensive mental hospital that takes care of people who are more severely demented. The point is, she would not be tried as a usual criminal, she would be tried as a mentally ill patient. So, if we did not treat Emily as a usual citizen and imprison her for what she has done because of her mental illness, why did we imprison Larry Nassar for abusing little girls in private, when those actions are what his mental illness was urging his mind to do? Perhaps we decided to label him as evil because it was easier than understanding why he did what he did.

As humans, we often view the world in a very right-or-wrong, black or white fashion. The point of that was, again, not to defend the criminal actions of a pedophile. It was, to instead, prove to you that in this very complex life, there is no such thing as black or white. There are truly only shades of grey. In other words, everything is circumstantial. Your moral conclusions are not accurate if you are not taking into account every detail of the specific situation. So, instead of sticking to our rigid mental rules of things that are good and things that are bad, keep this in mind. It is common, even healthy, to create your own imaginary line in your head that separates the good from the bad. In all honestly, that self-made line is what guides our everyday behavior and keeps us from doing harm to others. However, in the real world, when it comes to making judgments about other people's actions there is no clear existing line between good or bad. It all depends on circumstance, and these circumstances are often times ignored because of our own personal bias.

PERSONAL BIAS

"It is not at all hard to understand a person; it is only hard to listen without bias." -Chriss Jami

BIAS BLIND SPOT

The bias blind spot (also known as meta-bias) is the cognitive bias of recognizing the impact of biases on the judgement of others, while failing to see the impact of biases on one's own judgment. In simpler words, you may think that others are biased without being able to recognize that you are too. This is typical human nature. People generally are able to more easily point out the flaws in another person's thinking, while being able to put their own minds on a mental pedestal that thinks only logically, without involving emotions. Consider the current president of the United States, Donald Trump. Now, pretend you are a normal kid, that is into politics and enjoys the topic of psychology. You are a student who's family has always been die-hard Democratic, and you are a Muslim, and a Pakistani, and you think that Trump is a racist. Instead of pointing fingers at someone who you might think is a lunatic, you are doing your best to understand why someone you consider "crazy" thinks the way that he does. So, you research peer-reviewed articles, and you read scholarly books written by P.H.D professors on the specific topic of Donald Trump and you are now convinced that Trump is mentally ill, with Narcissistic Personality Disorder. You may have done the research right- you went through the articles, and you came to a conclusion that you would like to believe that you based solely on fact. But this may not be true. You approached the situation already believing that Trump is mentally ill, so you found information that looked pretty to you. Even if Trump does have Narcissistic Personality disorder, that is not the point. The point is, you think you are no longer biased in believing it, because the facts match up with your claim. However, you are still biased. You did not read a single article with medical proof that Donald Trump is a regular human being with no signs of mental illness. Your so-called "unbiased" claim that Donald Trump is mentally ill may not be able to constitute knowledge at the end of the day, if you failed to recognize all sides of the story in order to prove your claim beyond a shadow of a doubt.

"GOOD STORY" BIAS

The "good story" bias can be incredibly powerful. Sometimes, when we are attempting to think critically, we overestimate the probability of scenarios that make for a good story, since such scenarios will seem much more familiar and more "real". In other words, we are more likely to choose to believe a story because it sounds good, or it feels right. This is one of the most common flaws in the variety of mistakes people tend to make, and it is often times blamed on just simply human nature. We must take the time to stop blaming errors on 'human nature' when these errors are ones that can be corrected in order to result in a more intelligent society. Take religion, for example. Pretend you are a Christian, and the Bible has told you since you were a young child that angels exist, and are sometimes even on Earth to protect us. Pretend you work at Papa Johns, and you learn that someone wanted to rob you. The only reason they did not end up robbing you, and potentially hurting you or killing you, was because the back door was somehow locked that night, even though it normally never is. You believe that an angel must have come to protect you. Whether angels are real or not, is not the point. The point is you may just be believing this because this story sounds good, makes you feel protected, and that explanation looks pretty to you. You have no logical proof of your claim. Maybe a coworker just remembered to lock that door that night. You are more likely to believe the religious story that you already believe to be true, rather than sensibly considering all alternatives.

PRESENT/PRESENT BIAS

This is a bias that can consume your judgment to the point where it can ruin your relationships. Whether it is a marriage, petty friendship, or serious relationship, individuals tend to focus on what is there rather than considering what is not present. In order to think more critically, you should of course take into account everything that is in front of you, but to set yourself apart from others, try and consider factors that are nowhere to be found before you make a conclusion. Here is an example of present/present bias in action:

You were just thinking about your husband, and how much you love him. Five minutes later, he calls you. You decide that your love was truly meant to be, since you he called you right when you were thinking about him. By coming to this conclusion, you are probably failing to recognize the hundreds of times you thought about your husband and he did not call you. You are believing what you want to believe.

CONFIRMATION BIAS

Imagine you are phone calling your friend to come to your house to spend some time with you, but they are not answering. You quickly come to the conclusion that they are avoiding you, and they do not want to see you. You come to this conclusion while they are ignoring you. You receive a text message from them four hours later, that reads "I'm sorry I didn't see your call, I was busy".

You use this response to confirm what you already thought, and suddenly you have decided that your friend is lying. You are now angry, because you think that they are not busy, they just didn't want to see you, when in reality they could have been completely busy and not available to answer a phone call. You don't know, because you don't care, because you *wanted* to be angry. This unnecessary spiral of emotions exemplifies exactly what confirmation bias is. Confirmation Bias is the tendency to interpret new evidence as confirmation of one's existing beliefs or theories. Seeking out the information that suits you can result in making ineffective decisions, and in the situation with the friend, this could result in burning bridges for effectively no reason.

AVAILABILITY HEURISTIC

The availability heuristic is a mental shortcut that relies on immediate examples that come to a given person's mind when evaluating a specific topic, concept, method or decision. This shortcut pushes images, memories, or stories that are more memorable or vivid than general information to the top. To further help you understand, use September 11, 2001 as an example. The horrific terror attack that terrified a countless number of Americans stands out to all of us, not only because of the number of deaths but because of the way this country completely changed afterwards. Before this day, security was not as extensive as it is now. The hatred against Isis grew after this event, and there were also significant rises in Islamophobia in the United States. Human beings are motivated by fear, and a terror attack has fear embedded into its every second. Statistically, you are definitely more likely to be killed in a car accident than you are in a plane crash. So, why do human beings say prayers and worry when their loved ones are getting on a plane, but they let their children drive off to hang out with their friends every night with almost no worry or doubt in sight? The one plane crash that killed thousands of people was so vivid, it stood out to you, and now you overestimate the possibility of a plane crash, while also underestimating the possibility of a more realistic event, like a car crash, happening to you or those around you.

EVIL

Our mind plays various tricks on us. It is our jobs to stump them, before they stump us. Now we are aware that our definitions of good vs. bad may very likely be incredibly flawed. However, I am not discrediting the existence and prevalence of evil in this world. I want you to take the instance of the kidnapped boy from the beginning of the chapter. For the purpose of reiteration, here is a summary of what happened:

It is 1997 in Texas. The seemingly good neighbors- (whatever "good neighbors" means), the ones that don't make too much noise, that work jobs, have a few kids, plant flowers here and there, and live their own separate lives lose their child. One day, their youngest son, Nicholas, goes missing. He was only 8 years old, with beautiful blonde hair and spiking blue eyes.

I did not make this up. The true story of Nicholas Barclay was later turned into the infamous documentary titled "imposter." Here is the rest of the story, which describes all relevant instances that all occurred starting eight years after Nicholas goes missing:

A 16-year-old boy in Spain by the name of Frédéric Pierre Bourdin has lived in foster care systems his entire life, and wants a family and will go to any means to get one. He calls American police departments- the Florida Police department, the NYPD, and the Georgia Police Department, and collects research on all boys who went missing about eight years ago- so that they would be 16 (his age) now. His plan is to pretend he is that missing boy, so that he will receive a family that loves him. The boy he chose was Nicholas Barclay, who, if I may add, has blonde hair and blue eyes. Frédéric has brown hair, so he dyes his hair blonde and cannot do anything about the eye color. He also carries a thick Spanish accent- so this is not a believable lie, on any account. So, he lays in the middle of the street and a woman finds him, and asks if he is okay, but he doesn't respond. He wants the woman to believe he's senseless, and she does, so she calls the police. He lets the police know that he is Nicholas Barclay, and comes up with a kidnapping story. They send him back to America and the family, on camera in tears, accepts him with open arms, and seems to be genuinely thankful to have their son home after so many years.

An investigator becomes interested in the case. This boy does not even have an American accent, but the parents just quickly accepted him as their son and took him home. So, he digs, and this is what he finds:

Nicholas Barclay was killed by the parents when he was eight years old. Eventually, the kidnapping story died down and everyone forgot about it. However, when they got a call from the police that said someone had found their son in Spain, they had no choice but to pretend like they were happy he was home. So, these people kept this total stranger in their home as family to cover up their murder.

This may be a very extreme case, but I am simply pointing out the fakeness in things that seem all so genuine; surely, the most inexplicably horrific of deeds come from the most unexpected places. It is wise to live your life with an air of caution at all times. Truly, evil does exist and unfortunately, as with the parents of Nicholas Barclay you cannot always blame the acts that a person chooses to commit on a mental disorder, or unusual circumstance. Many times, people do evil things purely because they want to. In my opinion, the blackest and most extraordinarily wicked part of reality is comprehending that many times, it is the most seemingly genuine people that create the worst lies, or do the most horrible things. Most people in society are able to comprehend that people are not usually what they seem to be. This turns out to be one of the biggest lessons that teenager's learn as they are growing older. Truly, people show you only what they want you to see.

So, let's talk about the components in human nature that, once spiraled out of control, provide an entry-way for harmful behavior and a solid starting point for the evil that does exist in this world:

JEALOUSY

"You can be the moon, and still be jealous of the stars." - Gary Allan

The typical human is in denial of the envy that is embedded into our hearts. Jealousy can take on one of the most dangerous presences in our lives, and failure to control the ways we react to jealously pushes you in a corner that can leave you with very little respect from others. Habitually we learn that is it okay if other people are not happy for you. Then, we are generally comforted by being told that those same people, are most likely not happy with themselves. I cannot say that this applies to every case of every jealous person all of the time, but this sense of entitled insecurity is what drives a very high proportion of them, but not all of them. Here is an example in action of personal bias- surely, we as individuals are more likely to consider ourselves "not jealous people" than we are to categorize ourselves as "jealous people". Whether we want to admit it or not, we all do it, some more than others. Everyone, to some extent, is a jealous person because it is not something we have much control over. In truth, it is a natural, instinctive emotion that everyone experiences at one point or another. The uniqueness about jealousy is it normally takes the form of an extra external drive, to prove that you are better than somebody else. The stronger an individual's feelings of jealousy are, the more likely it is that that individual is simply using jealousy to protect his/her own deep-seated feelings of anger and obsessiveness.

Think in your mind of what jealousy feels like; someone else is happy or successful while we are left alone to overthink and compare ourselves to them. Take a form of jealousy that is most likely common to you: relationship jealousy. Your husbands' "first love" or your daughter's first boyfriend are not the intimidations we think they are. It is the overwhelming, obsessed state of cynicism we enter because of these people that may cause us to do things that can ruin a relationship, or a romance.

Think about the thoughts we have when we feel jealous. The fear of looking bad or losing reputation points drives us to be over-critical about our own lives. It is thoughts like, "why is my daughter not as innocent as hers?", or "why am I not as good-looking as him?", that may push us to express these emotions in extremely unhealthy and belittling ways. Now, all of a sudden, since your daughter is not as innocent as hers you may create gossip to your circle of friends about how "bad" the seemingly better one really is, just so that your party doesn't look so bad by comparison. Unhealthy. Now, since you are angry someone else looks better than you, you may spend money you don't have so that you can try and look more like him. Unhealthy.

Jealousy is a natural emotion that can be controlled. It is important to remember that your problems are almost 95% your mindset and 5% your actual problems, unless you are dealing with extenuating circumstances or a mental disorder. Collectively, our mindsets shape our actions and our actions shape who we are as a person.

Succumbing to jealous thoughts are what force us to commit to unwarranted behaviors. Sometimes so much, people may avoid you. Here are some questions to stop and ask yourself when you find yourself in a situation where you are jealous of someone else, and you find yourself showing aggression over those negative emotions, such as making up lies about the person:

1) Am I making excuses to myself to justify that they deserve to be talked about?
2) Do I have a valid reason to not like this person?
3) The qualities that I am pointing out as being "wrong" about this person, do I see any of those same qualities in myself?
4) If these people knew who I truly was under my social mask, would they still like me?
5) Am I acting in a way that makes me respect myself?

6) Am I acting in a way that makes others respect me?

Jealousy is normal, but once it spirals out of control it is a negative emotion that blatantly weighs down the heart. It sends your moral compass array. It is important to realize that in everyday life, if we choose to act on our feelings of jealousy instead of doing our best to maintain an internal balance between acceptance of what others have vs. acceptance of what you have, our true feelings may very easily show through. As you are reading this, you may feel as though this may not apply to you, but it applies to almost everybody, just in different ways. Jealousy will always be found even in the purest of hearts and proves to be a demon we are all meant to fight- we are simply in different levels of hell.

GOSSIP

"Sometimes, people try to expose what's wrong with you because they cannot handle what is right with you."
-Avinash Wandre

Gossip is jealousy's twin sister. Surely, backbiting is understood as one of the most normalized and also one of the most destructive evils in society. Whether we would like to admit it or not, for many individuals, the urge to expose negative details or adverse opinions about someone we are jealous of lies closer to us than our jugular vein. The next time you meet someone who lets you know that they "never gossip", do not be fooled. This is merely not true. Gossip is well-defined as the casual or unconstrained conversation or reports about other people, typically involving details that are not confirmed as being true. Frequently, when we think about gossip, we think about scattering lies or rumors that may not be true. However, this traditional form of attempting to ruin an enemies, or more often, a "friends'" social standing is not the only form that the evil of gossip takes place in. Talking about others is a habit that individuals may leech on to as young children- a habit that is not easy to break. In many social situations, it actually acts as a powerful instrument used to bond with those around us. Think about a time you had something juicy to talk about- a scandal, a divorce, you caught someone in a lie. Now, think about a time where you took this juicy information and used it in a group of people, or even just to one other person. More likely than not, it probably felt like you were saying, "hey, I'm giving you this information because you're important and this person I'm talking about isn't." Or, in some cases, it can be like saying, "I'm giving you this information (even though I know it may not be true) because it sounds interesting and in turn makes me a more interesting person." It can be a tool used to seem important, and an excuse to feel important.

Sometimes, it can be hard to tell if somebody is talking about someone else out of envy, or if they are just spreading facts about someone who is a bad person. Unfortunately, the typical human is manipulative enough to speak badly about someone without making it look like they are trying to push the person in a harmful light. In simpler terms, people tend to gossip about others while also pushing themselves in a more positive light. Here are some questions to ask yourself while attempting to evaluate the intentions of a gossiper:

1) Does the gossiper already have something against the person being gossiped about? (Try and find the history between the gossiper and the person being gossiped about. Are they old

best friends that had a falling out? Are they fighting for the love of the same person?)

2) Is the gossiper targeting uncontrollable factors about their looks or speech? ("she's ugly", "I've never seen someone more unattractive", "her lisp is so annoying!")

3) Is the gossiper being racist? (So, is the basis of their insults about the person's skin color, accent, or race?)

These three questions will assist you in your attempt to eliminate the act of blindly trusting the word of uncouth people. They are all more specific formats that beg the same general question:

Is the gossiper's hatred or dislike for the person irrational?

If the basis for hatred is not justified or rational, the gossiper is most likely filled with envy. You have a number of possible options that can help you avoid being exposed to a situation where somebody is deliberately being taunted. The best one would be to nicely to stand up for the person being talked about, even if you do not know them. If you do not want to do that, you can leave. Find better friends. Seemingly, taunting those we do not like behind their backs is extremely standardized in society, but that does not make it healthy. Gossip is a stab in the back. Rumors can socially isolate anyone, whether they are male or female. Once spiraled out of control, a buildup of events that start with gossip can result in higher rates of depression, suicide, eating disorders, and other mental disorders. Good words can move mountains, but bad ones can destroy people.

LYING

"Those who think it is permissible to tell white lies soon grow color-blind." -Austin O'Malley

Logically speaking, little white lies are simply ushers to larger black ones. For each seemingly "small" lie, the average person typically tells two more just to maintain the first lie. Lies destroy people, corporations, political parties, or clubs. Lies may serve as the basis for backbiting; they can also serve as the basis for jealousy. "Common sense" tells us that lying is wrong, when in reality, the same people that agree that lying is "wrong" would also agree that they use lies as a very powerful tool to provide oneself with an advantage in society. Lying is defined as the act of speaking falsely or utter untruth knowingly. According to psychologists in this era, a failure to speak (to deliberately withhold the truth) is also considered lying. Take the criminal justice system, for example. If our current president knew that a terrorist attack was going to occur in the United States and failed to say a single word, he would be tried in federal court and most likely would end up in prison. The failure to withhold evidence does not mean you did not lie. It is the failure to indicate whether somebody is deceiving us that ends up breaking hearts, ruining business deals, or, as in the example with the president, killing people or destroying lives. According to Pamela Meyer, rendered from her Ted Talk about lie detecting, studies show that you may be lied to between 10-200 times a day. When we hear this data, we recoil. We cannot believe that lying is so common. There is a popular belief that we lie more because we have to, than for fun. This is also not true. Studies show that we lie more to strangers than we do to coworkers or friends. Studies also show that we lie eight times more about ourselves than we do about other people. So, the prospect that humans are more likely to lie in a situation where they feel as if they are pushed to lie is simply inaccurate. Becoming a more experienced lie-spotter will assist you in avoiding the likely situation of being deceived.

Please note, that these are simply indicators. We are human beings- we make a various number of choices about our body language, eye movement, and so on every single day. Correlation does not prove causation- these things do not mean anything in of themselves. Instead, they are logical and scientific based indicators that point towards a liar. So, we will go over the criteria on how to indicate a person is a liar, starting with ways to catch somebody red-handed by their body language.

DETECTING A LIAR

BODY LANGUAGE

1) Many psychologists previously believed that you can tell if a person is lying by their eye movement. Common sense may tell you that "lying eyes" must be a thing, because surely, if someone is nervous about what they are saying it is going to be harder for them to look you in the eyes while they speak. Then, once you believe this, it is easy to find information that confirms your belief, which is yet another example of the way bias flaws our personal thought processes. If humans were as pure as we would theoretically like them to be, this could be proven true. However, this statement is unreliable because unfortunately *a liar is more likely to not feel guilty for telling a lie than he is to feel guilty.* Among the general population, this sense of nonchalantly telling a

lie without regret normally comes about when it is a lie that we justify as being "harmless". To vindicate my point, think of your teenage days. Why was it easier to lie to our parents than to lie to our friends? Because our parents were in the way of whatever we wanted- going out, staying out late, having a girlfriend or boyfriend, doing drugs. Think about your own feelings when you are telling a lie. You probably don't feel nervous. You honestly, deep down do not feel bad either. The sad truth of reality is that manipulation has become so common among society, we are more likely to feel bad for not feeling bad than we are to feel guilty for lying to people who love us. The common misconception is that if a person looks to the right, or the left, they are more likely to be lying than telling the truth. Contenders of this belief also point out that if a person can look you in the eyes and make a claim, they are probably telling the truth. This is a myth. The most stone-cold killers are able to lie to police without blinking or shifting eye movement. Why is that? Because they did not feel guilty, they just want to get away with what they did. To shift the perspective to an example that may be more relatable to you, imagine you are a teenager that is caught with drugs. If your parents find out, they will send you to boot camp, so you are afraid of them. This fear will drive you to be a better liar to protect yourself, even if you may not consider yourself a "bad person", or a typical liar.

There is no evidence of a correlation between lying and eye movements.

It is the hands, not the eyes. A person that is lying waves their hands around, and uses hand gestures to emphasize their innocence, far more than a person who is being honest. Here is an example of what that may look like to you:

SCENARIO: Denya is a 17-year-old girl. In her culture, it is strictly forbidden to have any contact with the opposite gender in a relationship-type way until she is married. In simpler terms, Denya is not allowed to have a boyfriend, and if she does, her parents will not respect her anymore. She decides to have a secret boyfriend regardless of the possible consequences. On Valentines Day, Denya goes out with him and lies to her parents about where she is- she says she is working late that day. Denya's parents go to her job to visit her, and she is not there.

Pretend you are Denya. Your parents are calling you, so you rush home. They are waiting for you, at the kitchen table, extremely angry and already assuming the worst. For a 17-year-old girl who is afraid to lose her parents respect and the ability to have freedom, this is a very high pressure situation.

Denya explains that she was with her friend Courtney. They were just at Starbucks, eating food. Note that Denya is aware she is lying: now her mind is begging the question- how does an innocent person talk? When her mom accuses her of having a boyfriend, Denya puts her hand on her forehead and rolls her eyes. "Mom, you're ridiculous, I would never do that." She does not want to seem nervous, so she is consciously attempting to act normal. She pushes her hair behind her ears while she speaks, then she rolls her sleeves up while she defends herself, and then she taps her own forehead or her chin or rubs her legs to make herself look natural and nonchalant. **It's in the hands.**

2) **Liars will blink more or less often than usual.**
3) **Liars may have a slight delightful expression while deceiving another, known as Duping Delight.**

You may often times notice somebody smiling when they are being questioned. Sometimes, the smile may be out of nervousness, or the increase in blood pressure. However, there are times where a person will smile once they have deceived someone. This is known as duping delight, and it is mostly noticed among criminals. Though it is not commonly detected in the usual population and is more noticed in the world of psychopaths and serial killers, once educated on the matter of spotting duping delight you may be a step closer to catching your liar. Here is an example:

LINE 1: Mom: Denya, do you have a boyfriend? You know you are not allowed.

LINE 2: Denya: (obviously lying) no, Mom. I don't. I would never disrespect you or Dad in such a way! It is ridiculous to think I would have a relationship with someone that is more than friends. I feel offended, honestly, that you think I would do something like that.

LINE 3: Mom: I am sorry for asking, sweetheart. Do not be offended. I love you, and I trust you!

In this scenario, you would look for an indication of duping delight during line three, or perhaps right afterwards. Denya has successfully deceived her mother, and even though Denya may not be a bad person, she is relieved that her mother believed her lie.

4) LEAKING EXPRESSIONS

You do not have to be a certified facial expression expert to know how to look for a leaking expression. After a first date that went awfully wrong, you may catch your date partner leak an expression of frustration through his/her regular smiling facial expression. Perhaps the date partner was so determined to let you know that he/she was unbothered, they had a very convincing mask of delight on. In another instance, suppose a murderer is being interviewed, and is letting the interviewer know that he is completely cold-hearted and does not regret killing anyone that he killed. You may, after a few minutes of conversation, catch the murderer leak an expression of sadness. Though this does not relate to a direct lie, leaking expressions relate to an individuals core feelings and is a valid method in attempting to understand what lies under a mask of charisma and smiles.

SPEECH:

1) When a liar is lying, they are more likely to resort to formal language than informal language. Example: Bill Clinton's affair with Monica Lewinsky. In an interview questioning Clinton about the affair, this was his response:

"I did not have sexual relations with that woman… Miss Lewinsky."

Formal language. The liar wants to sound more intelligent, which in turn, he thinks may make him sound more confident. He calls her "Miss

Lewinsky", instead of Monica. He sounds more detached from the situation.

2) Distancing language: A liar is very possibly going to use this tactic to verbally isolate themselves from the situation. Use the same example:

Bill Clinton: "I did not have sexual relations with that woman… Miss Lewinsky."

"That woman". He refers to her as "that woman", which makes her sound like someone he hardly knows. Then, he repeated her name after he said "that woman". This was done to show listeners that he may not know her very well at all. She is so irrelevant and unknown to him, she is just "that woman", instead of "Monica".

3) They will alter their vocal tone, often making their vocal tone much lower.

This lower tone is usually used by the liar to manipulate the listener into believing that he or she is genuine. Their logic is this: it is the kinder people that talk more calmly. Also, they think that people who are lying will be defensive, and defensive people will raise their voice. So, they are trying to sound like they are mature, well-put together, and more than anything else: sincere.

> 4) The liar will ask specific questions about the incident, person, or situation in question.

A liar will often times come up with questions to ask the person that is interrogating them. Here is what that may look like, with an example with John, who cheated on his wife.

John: Honey, why are you angry?

Wife: I know you've been cheating on me, John.

John: **Where did you hear this from?** That is simply not true!

Wife: Where I heard it from does not matter! I was told you slept with the neighbor Monica last week.

John: Last week! Absurd! **What day in specific did this ridiculous accusation supposedly take place?**

Wife: Tuesday. Tuesday night, but it really does not matter which day.

John: That is ridiculous. I was with the kids all of Tuesday night taking care of them while you were at work! You know this. I would never hurt you, you are my wife. **Now, who told you that this happened? Was it a friend?**

Notice the number of questions John asks to deflect the wifes' main question of him cheating. John's character is being attacked here, so he must deflect the attention elsewhere. Also, the questions assisted him in gaining a more specific view of the exact knowledge that his wife has come across, this way he can fit his lie to make some sense. Once he knows exactly when the accusation took place, he can desperately prove to her that he was not doing that on that day at that time. If he was innocent, he would likely have more vaguely said that he is not guilty, and he would care more about why his wife even believes such a rumor than the specifics of the incident.

Jealousy, gossip, and lying are all very natural human tendencies that serve as the basis of harmful behavior. These are not all the bases of harmful behavior; however, these are among the most common.

DETECTING A PSYCHOPATH

"We serial killers are your sons, we are your husbands, we are everywhere. And there will be more of your children dead tomorrow." -Ted Bundy

The DSM-5 (Diagnostic and Statistical Manual for Mental Disorders, most recent version) has given psychopathy the official title of Anti-Social Personality Disorder. The media often equates the word psychopath or sociopath to "serial killer". Take Ted Bundy, for example, America's most notorious serial killer who raped and murdered more than 30 women, and went undetected for years because he lived a seemingly "normal" life. Bundy was a brilliant psychopath to have gone unnoticed for so long- and his wicked weapon? Manipulation.

1) INSINCERE CHARM

"Psychopathic charm is not in the least shy, self-conscious, or afraid to say anything." Hervey M. Cleckley

Psychopaths are performers. They will say "I'm sorry" in the right sympathetic tone, or tell a woman they love them with the right amount of nervousness and connection in their eyes, while they lead them to their apartment to murder them. Consider Ted Bundy again. He was so charming and attractive, various women sent him marriage proposals even while he was on death row for raping and killing over 30 women. The superficial charm of a psychopath is among their strongest tools of manipulation, because it is characterized with a mix of deviant intelligence. Though it is superficial it looks extremely natural.

2) GRANDIOSE SELF-WORTH

A sense of grandiose self-worth simply means that you have a sense of extreme arrogance that tells you that you are better than everyone else. Similar to every other characteristic of a psychopath, this tone of egotism is driven by the need for power. You see this among a disturbingly high number of politicians and government officials. Many politicians desire the two things that a typical narcissist also desires: money and power.

3) PATHOLOGICAL LYING

A pathological liar is simply a convulsive liar. The stories they tell are usually astounding and interesting to listen to, but they never breach the limit of normality but they are still believable. This is their tactic. The stories that the liar tells are also most likely going to add up to present the psychopath in a pleasant way (heroic, intelligent, saint-like).

4) LACK OF REMORSE

Remorse is self-regret. A psychopath does not feel guilty for being harmful to another person where an average person who is not a psychopath might, but the key is a psychopath is good at faking it. They will manipulate their spouse with tears and an "I'm sorry", when really, they are not. A lack of remorse serves as the basis of any sort of explanation to a psychopaths actions; they kill, rape, murder, and deceive consciously because that is what they want to and they merely do not think twice about it.

5) INAPPROPRIATE SEXUAL BEHAVIOR

A psychopath is essentially motivated by power, which is indicated by the grandiose self-worth and is backed by a lack of remorse. A lack of remorse suggests they have a lack of emotional connection between themselves and others- this is why sex is never about emotions for them, it is about power, boosting their own ego, or making them feel on top. Many psychopaths result to sexual harassment, rape, or even inappropriate masturbation in public to relieve this need to feel as if they prevail over the "common" people.

For fun, here is a common question that psychologists may use to determine whether one is a psychopath or not:

A 27-year-old female teacher is teaching a first grade class at an Elementary school. A teenager with a gun enters the school and begins shooting students. As the teacher is frightened for her life, she turns off the lights in the room and locks the doors to protect the children. Eventually, someone opens the door. It is a man that she has never seen before- he is attractive, with wide shoulders and messy brown hair. He quickly and quietly directs the children out of the classroom and eventually out of the school. He saves their lives. Then, he helps the female teacher out, and she feels as if it is love at first sight. She is too shocked to ask him his name or number, and he leaves after kissing her on the cheek. She asks around to see if anyone knew who he was, so perhaps she could find him and talk to him but no one seems to be able to help her. A week later, she brings a gun to the school, and shoots five children. Why did she shoot up the school?

Try and answer this question on your own before you read the answer.

The "right" response:

If you asked this question to somebody and they were not psychopathic at all, nor did they have any violent or sociopathic tendencies (so, the average person in society) they would (most likely) provide you with one of two responses. The first one is that she shot up the school out of anger. Perhaps she was depressed or mentally ill and the frustration of not being able to find the man drove her off the edge so she decided to kill others in a way that was familiar to her, since the school shooting had happened just a week before. The second common guess is that the shock of the school shooting drove her insane and essentially "broke" her rational thought processes, for the purpose of simplicity and lack of a better term.

The psychopathic response:

If your response to this question was this, you are probably a manipulative person. The answer a psychopath would give is this: The woman shot and killed children in the school because the last time she saw him was at a school shooting, so it is likely that she will see him again at another school shooting. She wanted to see him again. See? The psychopath removed all emotions (like jealousy, hurt, and frustration) and focused solely on the goal of putting the woman into power. She wanted to see the man again, so she found a way.

Answering one question does not determine whether someone is a psychopath or not. It simply gives researchers, detectives or psychologists a more accurate feel of the inclinations of a person's mind.

DETECTING A THIEF

Becoming aware of what to look for in a stranger in order to assess if their intentions are genuine or not is one of the greatest shields against harmful behavior. The only robberies to protect yourself against are not the people who drain you emotionally- you also must consider the manipulative abilities of a stranger. Failure to detect or anticipate harmful behavior may result in a very dangerous circumstance. Here are the common practices of a thief, so you know what to look out for:

- CASING:

When premeditating a robbery at a department store, such as Nordstrom or Macy's, a thief will often times use the concept of casing. All this means is taking pictures of the inventory. You will generally see this in a form of selfies- a smiling man or woman will nonchalantly be taking many "selfies" around different areas in the fine jewelry department, but in reality they are pretending. They take pictures of the inventory and study it so that they have a better feel for the area before they strike.

- WAIT... WHY SO DEPENDENT ON ME?

When a thief is attempting to attack you personally and take your things, whether that be your wallet or the laptop in your car, they are likely to come up with a good crisis story first. For example, pretend you are walking to your car after class at the public University you attend. There are many people around, but one lady comes up to you and tells you that she cannot find her car and she really needs your help. She proceeds to ask you for a ride to the other parking deck to find her car. The first question to ask yourself is this: **why did this person approach me, and not security or the campus police officer?** In this situation, your best bet is to politely decline but offer to bring over a security officer or police man to help her find her car. This was the greatest indicator of her ill-intentions. A logical, genuine person would immediately look for a professional for help, not a random citizen. There is a reason we call 911 in an emergency when we need help instead of running to find a random neighbor in the street.

- APPEARANCE:

Often times, we trust that people who look poor (homeless, ratted clothing, uncombed hair, etc) are more likely to rob us than somebody with nice earrings and a professional outfit on. *This is how they deceive you.* You do not expect a wealthy looking woman with a nice purse to take advantage of you, so if someone with a beautiful appearance comes and asks you to let her sit in your car so that she can find hers, past experiences have told researchers that you are more likely to help even though the circumstance is the same. In modern times, it is actually more common for someone with diamond jewelry and brand-named get-up to rob you than it is for a homeless person. Chances are, the homeless person just wants five dollars from you, while the wealthy person wants a hundred.

A very unnoticed game that the human mind plays on individuals involves attractiveness. I will now accentuate the dangerousness of the dreaminess of beauty and charm, and the impact our inclination to attractive people has on our actions.

THE ILLUSION OF BEAUTY

We have all seen it happening before our eyes- the pretty girl gets all the attention, or the attractive man gets all the friends. An attractive girl may, for example, be able to be more easily forgiven for doing something wrong if she is able to bat her eyelashes and cry delicately, than someone who does not have very many eyelashes or tears. It is indebtedly true that an employer is more likely to hire you, or your fiancé is more likely to go through with marrying you if you are eye candy. Why do people tend to like attractive people more than they like unattractive people?

- THE "BEAUTIFUL IS GOOD" STEREOTYPE:

This stereotype just means that beautiful people are associated with good qualities. For example, if a girl you think is very beautiful donates 5$ to a homeless person, you will associate that girl with a good deed. Your thought process is likely to go like this: "wow, she is so pretty, and also so nice!". Whereas, imagine an unattractive person donates 5$ to the same homeless person. Your thought process is likely to be something like this: "They may be ugly, but they are nice." It is incredibly shallow but unfortunately, it is how our mind plays tricks on us. Now, the unattractive person is nice but you are still more inclined towards the attractive one that did the same good deed. It is true that in many (but not all) situations an unattractive person has to work twice as hard to be considered as "good" as the pretty one. In another example, take the simplicity of a smile. If a pretty girl who is a stranger to you smiles at you in public, you are likely to associate that action with kindness. If an older man with ratted clothing and an unattractive face smiles at you in public, you are likely to call them creepy.

- DECIEVING OUR PERCEPTION OF TIME

Just as every other concept in Psychology, this is not expected to explain every single case all of the time. It is, however, a valid explanation for a high proportion of people. It may seem ridiculous that the illusion of beauty may even differ your perception of time, but it is true. For example, think of a time you spent a day with a beautiful person. Chances are, you enjoyed looking at that person and you enjoyed their attention being completely on you so much you were not bored, even if this person was not the most interesting person in the world. In recent years, a study measured beauty's influence on time perception. Researchers found that when men spent an hour with somebody who they considered attractive, the time flew by. However, when men were paired with a woman that they did not find attractive, the time spent with them seemed to drag on. The saying "time flies by when you're having fun" seems to have some truth to it. The only thing that saying doesn't mention is the strong correlation between having a good time and being around an attractive person.

THE ILLUSION OF LOVE

You will notice that love does not always mean sex. There are many couples that do not have sex until marriage, and there are some couples that even stay without sex during marriage, though this is rare. You will also notice that love does not mean you have a bond with someone- sometimes, we find ourselves most distant from our partners when theoretically, they are the ones we should be closest to. Love does not mean commitment, either. Nor does it mean having a romantic relationship.

The definition of love is subjective, and must be defined operationally in every research experiment. Researchers must come up with criteria for what love means in their experiment, if that is what they are testing. There is no real definition of love. It means something different for every person. However, the idea of "love" manipulates our minds, whether our love is real or not.

If your leg is broken, you are less likely to consider if anyone around you also has a broken bone and you are more likely to focus on your pain. If you just got your dream job, you are less likely to think about all of the people who are unemployed and most likely to focus on your good news. Every powerful sensation or feeling causes us to focus more on what we feel, which in turn, lowers the extent to which we consider how others feel.

So, how does the overwhelming feeling of love affect our judgment?

- TURNING A BLIND EYE

The communal saying "love is blind" holds much veracity to it. It is commonly understood in psychology that people tend to look at a loved one through rose-tinted glasses. These rose-tinted glasses are usually the culprits when trying to find out why we tend to ignore the bad qualities of a person because we love a person so much. This is why a wife may not notice her husband's yellow, decaying teeth while he speaks because she loves what he is saying so much; alternatively, she does notice it, but she turns a blind eye. This is also why individuals defend their loved ones "bad" actions even if they are aimed at them themselves, such as cheating. The human mind has a habit of ignoring wrong behavior and focusing on the good as a mechanism of convincing ourselves that this person is worth loving.

- UNCONDITIONAL POSITIVE REGARD

Expecting an unconditional positive regard from your partner is one of the leading causes of failed relationships including marriages. This simply means that no matter what a person does, they expect to be regarded positively by their partner nonetheless. This is a flawed version of "love" that can be dangerous. For example, John's wife Susan expects an unconditional positive regard from him. She is incredibly rude to him at unwarranted times. She screams, and uses curse words. John is deeply bothered by her cursing and views this act of cursing disrespectful. Two hours after she insults him, she goes back to acting nice because she felt like it, and she assumes that he should be nice too because he loves her. This toxicity undermines Johns' feelings and pushes him into an unhealthy corner with barred walls. If you have anyone similar to Sarah in your life, it is very possible that you may notice that they get very offended when somebody else is offended by something they did, even if they were completely wrong.

- LOVE IS A DRUG

If you do not know what an emotion is, it is simply a product of a chemical reaction that happens inside of the human brain. A neurotransmitter (a transmitter neuron) is released whenever something happens, and eventually binds to another neuron that will inhibit or excite it. Within a few seconds, it will tell your brain whether what just happened was good or bad. The pleasurable and mind-fuzzing feeling that love, infatuation, attention, and sex give us are closely related to the feelings of taking a drug. When our partner (our source of love, infatuation, attention, or sex) leave us, we experience withdrawals. The absence of feeling wanted or the absence of an ego-boost after you have gotten used to it may force you to miss your former partner excessively, when really it is not the person you miss, but the feeling. I am not discrediting that true love exists, I am simply pointing out that "true love" and even happiness are merely emotions that are a product of the opiate-like reactions occurring inside your body. So, the longing for a person's "one true love" after they are gone may just be an individual manipulating themselves into believing that they miss the person and not the dopamine.

HOW TO MANIPULATE PEOPLE INTO LIKING YOU

Deception occurs in areas of our daily life- areas we may not even have realized existed. So, in a world full of con-artists and manipulative skill, we are probably putting up some sort of a mask in front of others, depending who they are. So, how should you go about convincing somebody that you are somebody worth liking?

1) MIRRORING:

Copy them. This does not mean you should copy the things they say word for word, nor does it mean you should take an interest in the things that they are interested in. However, take note of small behaviors. Do they open the door for other people? If so, you are with a well-mannered person. So, be well-mannered yourself. Throw away any trash you see on the ground, or give an extra nice "excuse me" to the man that you cut in front of so your target understands that you relate to their morals. Consequentially, if you are able to relate to something as personal as morals, they will feel closer to your personality.

2) MERE-EXPOSURE EFFECT

The mere-exposure effect states that people tend to like things or other people who are familiar to them. To make someone like you on a first date, bring them to a restaurant that has food that you know they are familiar with and talk about it. Or, hang around them more often. This is a tactic useful in the professional working world, that works almost every time. Even if the action is as slight as grabbing coffee from the employee lounge room at the same time every day, the more you place yourselves near another person, the more familiar they are with you, which leads to comfort. Now they like you more than they like the average person.

3) SPONTANEOUS TRAIT TRANSFERENCE

This phenomenon is rather simple but unbelievably powerful. People will associate the traits you attach to other people, with your personality. So, when you are with somebody else, compliment a stranger. This will result in the person you are attempting to impress to believe you are a nice person. Humans gather evidence by observation. It is much more effective to let somebody else watch how you behave with other people whom you do not know. Do you go out of your way with them? Are you doing the bare minimum, or are you extra nice? You will find throughout your life that most people who are not your immediate family form 30% of their opinion on you based on how you treat them, and 70% of their opinion on you based on how you treat others.

4) EMOTIONAL CONTAGION

Emotional contagion simply states that people can feel the emotions around them. Your chances of being liked rise exponentially higher if you seem like you are in a good mood. Then, your chances of being liked are even higher if it seems like you have been in a good mood since before you met with them. They will be more attracted to your personality if they feel as if your happiness is impermeable, even if it is not.

5) DO NOT BE AN OPEN BOOK!

Logically, it makes sense that perhaps if you share the dark details of your life- your stories about child abuse, your parents divorce, your financial struggles- an individual may feel closer to you because you are sharing with them personal details about your life. This is true; however, be careful when you place these personal details. If you are on a first date and you let the other person know what makes you cry at night, they are likely to consider you a drag or a possible liability. Keep in mind that everybody has issues. Yours are important, but during the first few weeks of knowing someone try to refrain from spilling the gory details. Then, once you do share your personal issues after it has been a while, they may be surprised. They will respect you more if they see that regardless of your life issues you are a such a happy person and you do not even complain. Don't be an open book.

A NOTE FROM THE AUTHOR

THE SECRETS TO HAPPINESS

WITHOUT MANIPULATION

1) REMEMBER THAT YOU CANNOT MAKE SOMEBODY APPRECIATE YOU. If they don't, they probably never will. Remember that there are some people in this world, for whom you could travel to the sky for, and bring down the moon as a gift for them, and they would still say, "why didn't you bring me the stars?"

2) REMEMBER TO GET OUT OF A TOXIC ENVIORNMENT. In Biology, you will learn that if an organism cannot adapt to its environment, *it changes its environment.* This is how it survives.

3) REMEMBER THAT MAKING OTHER PEOPLE LOOK BAD WILL NEVER MAKE YOU LOOK GOOD.
4) REMEMBER THAT IF YOU HELP OTHER PEOPLE YOU WILL NEVER LIVE A TRULY SAD LIFE, REGARDLESS OF CIRCUMSTANCE. Psychologically speaking, if you do your very best to help out anyone, you will feel better about yourself, thus humbling you. Chances are your self-esteem will be incredibly hard to tear down if you build yourself to be a kind person.
5) REMEMBER THAT EVEN A SMILE IS A CHARITY. You do not need to be wealthy, famous or powerful to change someone else's life for the better.
6) REMEMBER TO BE HAPPY, LIKE A CHILD. Be happy for no reason, because if you are happy

for a reason, you are in trouble because that reason can be taken from you.

7) REMEMBER TO SPEAK KINDLY TO YOURSELF. Believe it or not, self-esteem relies heavily on words, not just feelings. If you look at yourself in the mirror and feel unattractive, tell yourself out loud that you have seen worse. If you wouldn't say it to a friend, don't say it to yourself.

8) REMEMBER TO COLLECT MOMENTS, NOT THINGS. Everyone that wants to be rich and famous, becomes rich and famous and eventually finds that it is not the answer.

9) REMEMBER TO CHECK YOURSELF. Keep a piece of paper, or a note on your phone. Commit yourself to doing one nice thing for a stranger every single day, even if that just means smiling

at someone. You will feel the results in your heart.

10) REMEMBER TO HAVE HOPE THAT GOOD WILL ALWAYS TRUMP EVIL. In any world crisis, you will always find groups of people helping. Do not let the media, or anyone else fool you. For every one handful of bad people there exists two handfuls of good people. Pride yourself, that even if the rest of the world does not agree, you still see the world as this beautiful place, because it is one.

AND MOST IMPORTANTLY...

11) REMEMBER TO PUT YOUR LIFE INTO PERSPECTIVE.

Your problems are 95% your mindset and 5% your actual problems. So, the next time you are eating a piece of pizza remember that there is a child out there somewhere that would do anything just to have the crust of it. The next time you are angry because your father scolded you, remember that there is an orphan child out there somewhere that would give anything just to hear his father scold him, because it would mean he is alive. And the next time you wake up in the morning, make sure to enjoy the moment because every day there are thousands of people who never do. This life is brutal, but this life is also very beautiful.

As J.K. Rowling states...

"Happiness can be found even in the darkest of times, if one only remembers to turn on the light."

REFERENCES

"Child of Rage Sovraštvo." Come 2 Film, 1997.

"On the case of faith…" American Psychological Association, American Psychological Association, www.apa.org/rss/.

https://www.thinkingfaith.org/articles/20130611_1.html

On Catharsis: *Bushman's Study Conducted in 2002: Does Venting Anger Feed or Extinguish the Flames? (Brad J. Bushman, Iowa State University)*

How many mentally ill people actually commit crimes: American Psychological Association: http://www.apa.org/news/press/releases/2014/04/mental-illness-crime.aspx

On women that abuse men: https://ncadv.org/statistics

On women that abuse men… The National Intimate Partner and Sexual Violence Survey:

https://www.cdc.gov/violenceprevention/nisvs/index.html

"Imagine you are in a 1997 world..." The bizarre story of Nicholas Barclay: https://www.theodysseyonline.com/the-mystery-of-nicholas-barclay

Why bad things happen to good people... https://www.psychologytoday.com/blog/broken-hearts/201001/why-do-good-things-happen-bad-people-and-how-not-be-bicycle

"Defending" the actions of a pedophile... The Larry Nassar Sexual Harassment Case: https://www.nytimes.com/2018/01/25/sports/larry-nassar-gymnastics-abuse.html

On defining pedophilia and Schizophrenia... DSM-5: DSM-5, www.psychiatry.org/psychiatrists/practice/dsm.

On defining the availability heuristic.. https://www.alleydog.com/glossary/definition.php?term=Availability+Heuristic

On how to detect a liar, information derived and example of Bill Clinton interview from the Ted Talk: How to Spot a Liar: Meyer, Pamela. "How to Spot a Liar." TED: Ideas Worth Spreading, www.ted.com/talks/pamela_meyer_how_to_spot_a_liar.

On characteristics of a psychopath and the example of the woman at her sister's funeral: The wisdom of Psychopaths written by Kevin Dutton: Dutton,

Kevin. The Wisdom of Psychopaths: What Saints, Spies, and Serial Killers Can Teach Us about Success. Scientific American / Farrar, Straus and Giroux, 2013.

On the illusion of beauty...
https://www.psychologytoday.com/blog/it-s-man-s-and-woman-s-world/201403/is-beauty-in-the-eye-the-beholder

www.ingramcontent.com/pod-product-compliance
Lightning Source LLC
Chambersburg PA
CBHW070151230526
45471CB00002B/611